Legal & Disclaimer

The information contained in this book is not designed to replace or take the place of any form of medication or professional medical advice. The information in this book has been provided for educational and entertainment purposes only.

The information contained in this book has been compiled from sources deemed reliable, and it is accurate to the best of the Author's knowledge. However, the Author cannot guarantee its accuracy and validity so cannot be held liable for any errors or omissions. Changes are periodically made to this book. You must consult your doctor or get professional medical advice before using any of the suggested remedies, techniques, or information in this book.

Upon using the information contained in this book, you agree to hold harmless the Author from and against any damages, costs and expenses, including any legal fees, potentially resulting from the application of any of the information provided by this guide. This disclaimer applies to any damages or injury caused by the use and application, whether directly or indirectly, of any advice or information presented, whether for breach of contract, tort, negligence, personal injury, criminal intent, or under any other cause of action.

You agree to accept all the risks of using the information presented inside this book. You need to consult a professional medical practitioner in order to ensure you are both able & healthy enough to participate in this program.

I0424964

Contents

Introduction

Do you suffer excruciating pain during your menstrual period? How about bones that feel like cracking with sudden moves? Do the nights appear to be so warm that you experience hot flashes? Do your genitals feel dry and your breast tender? Has digestion become a regular dilemma? Do you alternately suffer the opposing constipation and diarrhea? Does acne become your regular companion just before or during menstruation? If you experience any, most, or all these symptoms, chances are, you are suffering from hormonal imbalance. While these challenges have beset the female populace around the globe, the aftermath of these manifestations had varying levels of inconvenience that have made women ask, "Why me?" So without sounding like an empathic 911 dispatcher, don't worry because help is on its way.

Chapter 1 - The Traffic Signals Which Assure Our Body is Running Smoothly and Efficiently

Imagine traffic signals majestically suspended by industrial cords or dead-bolted on sturdy posts that are strategically situated at road intersections with their usual green, yellow, and red lights. These signaling devices moderate the flow of vehicles at any given time and at any given day. They direct motorists if they should proceed, slow down, or stop in systematic rhythm to ensure the smooth flow of traffic. Hormones are like traffic signals and your body is an infinite amalgamation of cross-road-like processes from the most basic needs, like hunger, to the complex systems, such as reproduction. Just like a well-maintained traffic light that is programmed to flash the appropriate light so vehicles wouldn't accidentally crash into one another, a well-balanced hormonal system secretes chemical messengers that regulate most of the major bodily functions, even your moods and emotions.

But how do you know that your internal cross roads are running smoothly and efficiently? Since your body has diverse hormonal secretions, understanding how your internal messengers function would give you a better grasp on aiding its play in your overall health and well-being. When you feel hungry and satisfy the need without binging, then your body system is at its optimal state. If your red-calendar date doesn't make you cringe in anticipation, you may sit back and relax. Physical activities that make you bend don't cause you to contort in pain? Give yourself a pat in the back! Do your nights allow you deep slumber without involuntarily waking up drenched in sweat despite enough ventilation? Hurray! When your anatomical parts that define you as a woman are reminders of your essence and don't cause you discomfort, you are on the right track. And if your eating habits don't cause you indigestion, diarrhea, or constipation, your hormones are all in place.

A well-balanced hormonal system is like a sail that gently propels a boat. It aids your body to function with minimal bumps. But life is also a bed of roses – with its accompanying thorns. These bumps and thorns, even if minimal, may cause some grave and life-changing inconveniences if left unaddressed. So for women all over the globe, a greater understanding of the major chemical messengers would go a long way.

3 Most Concern Hormones Which Promote the Healthy Development of Female Sex Characteristics

Estrogen

Estrogen, or estradiol, is what would be considered as the main female sex hormone. Produced by your ovaries, adrenal gland, and, although in minimal quantities, by your body fat, it assists in retaining the calcium in your bones. Remember those physical activities that give you a cracking-like feeling in your bones? A diminished level of estrogen is the culprit. The right level of estrogen in your body would balance out your high-density lipoprotein, or HDL (referred as the 'good cholesterol' that carries cholesterol from other parts of your body back to the liver for excretion), and low-density lipoprotein, or LDL (called the 'bad cholesterol' because its causes cholesterol buildup in your arteries when its level is high). If you find yourself high risk of acquiring diabetes or currently facing this dilemma, your estrogen level is something you might want to get a quick look at since estrogen assists in the maintenance of your blood-sugar levels. Finding trouble with memory retention or experience whiplash with your emotional ironies? Estrogen affects those, too. This hormone also triggers your puberty stage. It likewise is the front-line warrior that readies your body and uterus in the event of a pregnancy. Your menstrual period is regulated by this same hormone. Even when you reach the last hurrah of your propagation capability, the inevitable change in your estrogen level would greatly affect your experience as a woman as you progress in life.

Progesterone

While progesterone has similarities with estrogen, it isn't considered as the main sex hormone. Its level, however, plays an equally vital role when you experience your monthly cycle, as well as your 9-month period of nurturing a precious being inside your womb. It ensures that your uterus is up and ready for the fertilized egg nestling within. Have you been in various diet regimens to keep a sultry figure or aim for one? Progesterone helps in reducing your body fat and makes you worry less because it also aids in relaxation and reduces your anxiety of whether you'd reach your targeted body mass. Do you think you shed more than the usual hair when you hit the showers? Check out your progesterone level because it rejuvenates your hair follicles to induce growth for lustrous locks of flowing hair.

Oestrogen

Did you know that the hormone testosterone isn't purely male-defined? While it basically is the principal male sex hormone, you also produce a small amount of this chemical within your ovaries and adrenal glands. Just like testosterone, oestrogen is also common across both genders, but it influences the females more. As one of your main sex hormones, like estrogen, it plays a great role during your puberty stage and calcium enhancement that strengthens your bones. But then, everything in moderation, right? Too much or too little oestrogen would spawn a great deal of medical conditions that may be far worse than dysmenorrhea. What is equally important is that this chemical has a say as to how your brain synapses spark, the drum rolls of your heart, and flawless skin that every woman yearns for.

The Causes of Changes to our Delicate Chemistry Body

Weight gain, water retention, bloating – can you relate? These are but some of the effects of having too much estrogen, a medical condition referred to as Estrogen Dominance. Sad as it may seem, as women age, there is an innate downhill in your testosterone and progesterone levels, which leaves your estrogen levels to jump for joy as it remains in the limelight of your hormonal system. While predominantly, pre-menopausal women with a high level of estrogen bear the pear-shaped body due to the concentration of weight at the hips, when you reach your menopausal stage, the pear turns to an apple as the fat accumulation move to your abdominal area.

"Why on Earth would my estrogen level shoot up when I'm not yet menopausal?" you ask. There are two ways. One is innate while the other may be acquired. The 'built-in' part is when your body produces too much estrogen on its own. So, unless you could reprimand your hormonal system and command it to shut down its production of estrogen, this is pretty much something beyond your control. Also, if you already have health problems like obesity, ovarian tumors, or liver disease, these could easily raise your estrogen levels. The second way, however, is more controllable because increased estrogen levels could be acquired from your environment or diet. I can assure you that peaking your estrogen level is way too easy without putting any extra effort at all. Why? Because you are always in contact with estrogen-like substances that you find in food grown with pesticides, herbicides, and growth hormones. Whether the producers of these products admit it or not, these toxin-infused chemicals tip your weighing scale. Like a domino, your accumulated fat cells as you gain weight would further fuel your estrogen production into high gear.

Estrogen dominance may also arise if your progesterone level is low, which usually happens when you are under a lot of stress. If you live a stressful life, your progesterone and the stress hormone cortisol become the less priority of pregnenolone – the substance from which the two are formed. Now, what does that have to do with your increased estrogen? You see, when you are stressed, your body prioritizes your stress response and ignores your other body functions. So, instead of creating progesterone, pregnenolone makes more of cortisol to even out your stress. By doing so, less progesterone is produced and this tips your hormonal balance, giving estrogen dominance in your system.

When your detoxification is impaired, you are likely to have excessive estrogen in your body. Allow me to introduce you to your chemical factory – your liver. It carries so many tasks: filtering blood from your intestine, removing excess food and iron for future use, and destroys poisons and worn-out blood cells in your body. It also creates chemicals crucial to your system. Now imagine that your liver exhausted from all of those tasks and overburdened with many toxins. Instead of flushing out your excess estrogen, it gets recirculated back into your bloodstream. Estrogen is quite a persistent and stubborn hormone. It would keep on circulating until excreted through your feces. Since one of estrogen dominant effects is constipation, estrogen would be reabsorbed by your body and recirculated over and over.

Don't forget about the pharmaceutical hormones, like those used in hormone-replacement therapy (HRT). There are other medications that could increase your estrogen levels such as hormonal contraceptives, some antibiotics, herbal or natural remedies, and phenothiazines, a doctor-prescribed medication for some mental or emotional disorders. Estrogen dominance may also be gene-related; it runs in the family. So, whether you consume them consciously or you are unaware of when they make their way into the water that you drink, you are like a fish swimming in a vast sea of harmful estrogens.

While estrogen is both produced by the male and female bodies, having high levels of said hormone affects either genders differently. Unfortunately, the female-dreaded weight gain tops the list for women. But most of the time, those unwanted love handles choose to focus around the hips and what should have been an indented waist. As if your monthly cycle isn't uncomfortable enough, heightened estrogen will make you question why the males are spared from such an agony.

You think the causes of estrogen dominance above was a long one? Well, there's more. Please don't think that I'm trying to overwhelm you. I believe that it's best you're aware of the contributing factors to estrogen dominance because an ounce of prevention is better than a pound of cure. Now, what are the factors that trigger estrogen dominance?

Excess body fat – If it's more than 28%, then you are aligning yourself to estrogen dominance. This is common for post-menopausal women because estrogen is made in the fat cells. So, more fat cells equal more estrogen.

A low-fiber diet – If you consume too much carbohydrates, sugar, and processed food, you're not getting enough nutrients and high-quality fat (yes, you need fat too, but the good ones) into your body that may lead to a depleted magnesium level. Magnesium is the mineral that supports bone structure. Less of it would make your bones brittle, another effect of estrogen dominance.

Too much coffee – Who doesn't like coffee? But everything should be in moderation. Caffeine had been known to relate to higher estrogen levels. Research says that if you consume about four or five coffee cups daily, that's a whopping 70% more estrogen than those women who only have less than a cup.

Trans-fats - Do you love margarines? Then you might want to stay away from them. Margarines, as well as full or partially hydrogenated oils, are building blocks for hormones.

Nutritional deficiencies – Magnesium, zinc, copper, and B complex vitamins are crucial to neutralize estrogen in the liver. Deficiency of these vitamins would allow the estrogen in your system to proliferate.

Liver diseases – Remember your chemical factory mentioned above? Aside from being overworked with toxins, excessive alcohol intake that causes cirrhosis greatly reduce the liver's capability to breakdown your estrogen.

Signs and Symptoms of Estrogen Dominance

The accompanying symptoms of estrogen dominance vary between the sexes. For women, how would you know if your estrogen level is precariously hitting the scale even before having it checked? If you've hit your premenopausal stage, it's more than likely that you have the unwanted body fats around your hips. If you're still menstruating, its innate inconvenience could be coupled by irregularity, light to heavy bleeding, and heightened PMS symptoms.

Do these sound familiar – feeling bloated, having cold hands and feet, sleep deprivation, getting easily tired, losing hair more than usual, throbbing headaches, lessened interest in intimacy, mood swings, depression, anxiety, lapses in memory, allergies or food intolerance, gut permeability, and insulin resistance. While seemingly negligent and common, these are also the signs and symptoms of estrogen dominance. You may also find it difficult to lose weight despite your rigorous trips to the gym or sweat-inducing home exercises over stationary bikes. It's possible that you have a history of gallstone, varicose veins, uterine fibroids, cervical dysplasia, endometriosis, or ovarian cysts. And since estrogen imbalance is believed to be the cause of most cancers, it could be one of the main causes of breast and uterine cancer. The list of complications arising from estrogen dominance may even extend to thyroid diseases, salt and fluid retention, sluggish metabolism, infertility, blood clots, autoimmune disorders, accelerated aging process, heart attack, stroke, breast cancer, uterine cancer, and ovarian cancer.

Chapter 2 – The 6,000-Year-Old Alternative Medicine

You may find yourself saying one or some of the following:

"I am experiencing the symptoms."

"I consulted with a physician and was diagnosed to have estrogen dominance."

"I'm not experiencing any of the signs, but I'm nearing my menopause stage."

"I haven't experienced the symptoms, but I'm exposed to the triggers."

So, what should be your next step?

Essential Oils

Essential oils that help address estrogen dominance proliferate the world wide web. In fact, these oils have been used for thousands of years in a great diversity of cultures for both medicinal and health purposes. Essential oils have been used as antidepressants, stimulant, detoxifier, antibacterial, antiviral, and stress reliever. Of recent years, these oils became popular as naturally safe and budget-saving remedies for several health dilemmas and with the ever-climbing cost of healthcare bills, not to mention the accompanying possibility of side effects brought by conventional medicine, having essential oils as common items in your medicine cabinet would go a long way. Essential oils are like the jack-of-all-trades because of its bountiful benefits for a wide range of purpose that includes aromatherapy, household cleaning products, personal beauty care, and natural medicine treatments. There are those that support your liver to mobilize estrogen by applying it over the liver that is on the right side of your body and under your breast. Some remedies target the adrenal glands to regulate stress-resolving cortisol. You may even find some that focuses on your hypothalamus, the control center of the entire endocrine system that hormones are a part of. Another human anatomy that essential oils look at is your gallbladder. Since estrogen dominance turns your gallbladder bile too thick, rendering its efficiency to detoxify excess hormones less, essential oils working on your gallbladder would help mobilize your body toxins out.

What exactly are essential oils?

At one point in your life, you may have been given flowers, and most of the time, that would have been a rose. Remember how its scent pleased your olfactory sense? That was your pleasurable encounter with the aromatic qualities of essential oils. What gives the rose that distinctive aroma? It's in the seeds, bark, stems, roots, and the flower itself. While these essential oils give each flower a distinctive smell, it also protects the plant and aids in its propagation through pollination. But essential oils aren't just to please your sense of smell or ensure a plant's survival. History abounds with its use in the preparation of food, in enhancement of one's beauty, and practices that promote health.

Essential oils are volatile. It means that they easily change from a solid or liquid state into a gas, even in normal room temperature. Try opening a bottle of essential oil. You would immediately smell the potency of its aroma, even from a distance. Its volatile state disperses its scent easily through the air and instantly connects with your olfactory sense. Because of this unique property, essential oils have been integrated with aromatherapy solutions that help maintain a healthy mind and body. These essential oils have been leveraged even in emotional and physical wellness applications. Either as a single essence or a complex combination of blends, essential oils have accorded unique user experiences and a variety of benefits to people like you.

There are over 3,000 aromatic essential oils in existence as of today. Their essences vary from one plant to another, but the most important aspect is the precise ratio of the inclusive substances in the creation of essential oils. The ratio determines its efficacy in providing the specific benefits that you need. For essential oils to maximize efficacy, there are factors other than the composition ratio that must be taken into consideration. This includes the time of day, the season, the geographical location, the process and longevity of distillation, the year the plant was grown, and the weather. Each stage in the creation of essential oils is crucial to ensure that the end-product is of optimal quality, equally giving the benefits a boost to address specific areas of purpose.

Essential Oils for Estrogen Dominance

Your estrogen dominance is a feat on its own, so don't jump the gun and grab just any remedy. You must be very critical with your choice because hormone-mimicking elements, even essential oils, that enter your body may put you in a worse condition than you already are. As it is, you already have a system overload of estrogen and your liver already is in hyperdrive, flushing the excessive hormone out of your body. Remember, your body is already producing a lot of estrogen and aided by your fat cells that are burned, therefore, releasing more estrogen into your system. Of course, don't forget those you ingest through the food you eat, the beauty products that you use, and the environment that you live in. You wouldn't want to unconsciously feed your body more estrogen by using essential oils laden with estrogen-mimicking substances.

Essential oils can be rubbed on different areas of your body and since these oils have relatively small molecules, they can be absorbed by your skin to leverage the full extent of their effect. There are several essential oils known to balance and support your hormonal system. Rose essential oil, while known to be an aphrodisiac, is a natural mood lifter, a possible combatant for depression. It improves your serotonin, which is commonly known as your 'good-mood' hormone. Lavender and chamomile oils are also effective in stress reduction. When de-stressed, your cortisol levels are naturally low. This is very crucial, especially when your body is fighting off a disease.

The Help for Female Reproductive System to Return Balance

There is a long list of essential oils that generally improves your body and health. There are those that specifically stimulate your sex drive, reduce inflammation, improve your mood, remedy PMS cramps, reduce stress, and of course, balance your hormonal system. These oils help balance your estrogen level, which can improve conditions such as infertility, PMS, and menopause symptoms. In a 2017 neuro-endocrinology publication, certain essential oils were identified as influencing the salivary concentration of estrogen in women. So if you are experiencing menopausal symptoms due to a decline of your estrogen secretion, these essential oils would prove to be very helpful for you.

A lot of women have had great success in leveraging essential oils for hormonal imbalance and its accompanying symptoms. If you use these oils topically or diluted, these could be a helpful assistant as you struggle with PMS and other hormone-related illnesses that present themselves as you age. Some women prefer to use essential oils topically or aromatically because of the essential oils' inherent potency. When diluted, you reduce the risk of allergic reactions among other untoward incidents that may occur if the essential oil is undiluted or ingested. It would be crucial for you to seek a medical practitioner's opinion before using many of these essential oils, especially during pregnancy. This is because some essential oils can cause uterine contractions and cramping, conditions that could prove to be detrimental if you are pregnant.

Clary Sage Oil (Salvia Sclerae)

Referred to as, "the best oil for your worst time of the month," clary sage oil is a must-have for a woman like you. It is so powerful that merely inhaling its essence from the bottle could reduce your cortisol level. Whenever you feel that your stress level is running high, especially when you're nearing your menstrual cycle, reach out for your medicine cabinet clary sage oil bottle and sniff your stress away. Without sounding like I'm coaching you to act like a person hooked on a substance, immediately grabbing your indispensable bottle of clary sage oil has a beneficial purpose. A 2014 study on 22 post-menopausal women in their 50's reduced their cortisol levels and improved their thyroid hormones. The hero – Clary Sage Oil. The test subjects were initially diagnosed with depression, and after the trial period, the study showed that the clary sage oil acted like an antidepressant for these women. What's gives clary sage oil a frontline seat in terms of estrogen dominance? It helps with balancing out the estrogen production in your body. Since depression-induced stress triggers estrogen dominance, this essential oil would consequently lessen the production of estrogen in your system by reducing your stressing. When used for an abdominal massage, it could relieve that tightening feeling that is brought on by your menstrual cramps, as well as the discomfort due to the tension of your monthly period as the oil relaxes your smooth muscles. If you're searching for natural remedies for your PMS cramps or other high-estrogen-induced illnesses, look for the label that contains clary sage oil. This oil is such a powerhouse that most of the big companies carrying essential oil products almost always include clary sage as their primary oil to address PMS and hormonal imbalances in women. It greatly alleviates pain brought by PMS, reduces your stress, and improves your hormonal imbalance – the very culprit of PMS and menstrual problems.

Now, how does clary sage oil perform its magic? It has a unique hormone-like substance that balances out the estrogen production in your body. As a result, clary sage oil reduces PMS, menstrual cramps, and is quite effective in relieving pain, even in childbirth. Without sounding redundant, if you are pregnant, always be sure to consult your healthcare practitioner first.

Citrus Oils

It's crucial that you know this, but almost ALL essential oils have some levels of phytoestrogen. The good news is that citrus oils almost don't. So, make sure you check the label when getting your fix of lotions, shampoos, and deodorants. Lemon, lime, mandarin, and orange have almost negligible levels of phytoestrogens. Put these citrus oils on the top of your list. The best part about citrus oil, lemon in particular, is that it's liver-friendly. Lemon aids the liver in restoring full function to flush out the extra estrogen. Even a Dutch study determined that the compounds found in lemon peels, from which a substantial amount of lemon essential oil is extracted, aids in the improvement of liver function. It regulates your hormonal system by lowering liver cholesterol. Do stay away from tea tree, lavender, cinnamon, and peppermint. These have very high phytoestrogen content. Lemongrass is another variation and is sometimes referred to as a citrus sleep aid. Primarily, essential oils deal with hormones related to women, but lemongrass' fabulous scent pleases both genders' olfactory nerves. But more than just its scent, this oil would be a good friend to have close by because its power is to release your serotonin, the hormone that controls your mood, appetite, sleep, and even your cognitive functions. Just like other essential oils, lemongrass regulates your cortisol levels by relieving your anxiety. So, if you often have trouble sleeping, have eating disorder, or find it hard to concentrate, lemongrass is your best buddy. Its earthy smell has a hint of citrus that would be the number one choice for those who enjoy the scent of light lemon's freshness. As a precaution, be aware that lemongrass may have the tendency to irritate your skin. To avoid this, make sure you dilute the oil well enough and do a spot check beforehand. Just like the other essential oils, don't use it if you're pregnant unless directed by your health practitioner. Another 'no' would be to apply the oil compound near your eyes. Lemongrass blends well with essential oils such as jasmine, basil, and geranium. Here's another citrus variation. Would you like to say goodbye to your PMS symptoms? Allow me to introduce Melissa, also known as lemon balm oil because of its citrus-like scent. Melissa isn't heard of that often, but it is soothing when you apply it topically – that's why it's referred to as a balm. As an ally for your hormonal imbalance, its scent would be good company to keep right before your menstruation, when things get annoying and achy. It was a study in 2015 that gave this essential oil an efficacy in relieving symptoms of PMS. Aside from that, Melissa is known to boost your memory and combat fatigue and headaches. If you're a fan of citrus scents and you're suffering from PMS, take a look at this essential oil. Melissa may blend well with geranium, rose, and ylang-ylang. Another oil for citrus fans is Neroli, which is often referred to as the postmenopausal reprieve. This oil is extracted from the flowers of the citrus plant Neroli. In a study from 2014, it was concluded that when Neroli oil is inhaled by postmenopausal women, their symptoms were relieved. Here's another great effect: Neroli oil tends to ignite your sexual desire while dropping your stress levels. Who wouldn't want that, right? Of course, Neroli has other conducive effects. It eases your depression, kills bacteria in your body and even promotes the production of new cells from your head to your toes. But if you're a fan of the citrus family like orange, lemon and bergamot, you should avoid the sun so you won't have the phototoxicity issues inherent to citrus extracts. Equally important is that Neroli is a strong sedative, so if you need to stay awake, you might want to defer using this essential oil. It blends well with lavender, rosemary, and sandalwood.

Thyme Oil (Thymus Vulgaris)

Research found thyme oil's essentiality in balancing your progesterone levels all thanks to its phytoestrogen content, and since progesterone is an active player in your menstrual cycle by prepping your uterus lining for the possible implant of a fertilized egg, the balancing elements of thyme oil keeps your stress level in check. Aside from this, it eases the symptoms related to low progesterone such as alternating moods, sleep deprivation, warm feeling, and increase in weight. Earlier in this e-book, you've learned that a low level of progesterone gives an opportunity for your estrogen to rise. By leveraging it's benefit, you improve your progesterone production and inhibit your estrogen to monopolize your hormone system. This oil naturally balances out the hormones in your body. Besides, it is far better than resorting to synthetic treatments such as hormone-replacement therapy. Prescription drugs could make you dependent on them, possibly mask the symptoms that could hide what ails you, may have you developing diseases on other parts of your body, and probably cause some serious side effects. Thyme oil is also known to support your healthy immune system, consequently balancing your body system. This oil, just like rosemary, is an hereby oil that would provide you with a wide array of hormonal balancing benefits. Readily available if thyme is a staple in your medicine cabinet, this oil would be a handy companion if you are experiencing premature menopause or have blocked or painful menstruation because it could regulate your monthly cycle. Other benefits that you can get from thyme are relief from stress and alleviated depression, fatigue, and nausea. And since thyme is known to stimulate the production of your progesterone, this essential oil may kick those sticky estrogen in your system that seem to proliferate if you're in your menopausal period. Thyme blends well with bergamot, lavender, and rosemary.

Chapter 3 – Solution on the Horizon

Now is the time to breathe and relax because the solution to your problem of having too much estrogen in your system is right at your fingertips, or eye-level in the case of this e-book. The list of potent essential oils for hormonal imbalance is quite an extensive one, but what you find below will give you a substantial idea on how this miracle oil works and the magic it could do in the tipped off balance of your hormonal system.

The Miracle Methods

There are specific essential oil application procedures that are designated for certain ailments that women just like you suffer from that is brought on by your estrogen dominance. But with continuous research, several application methods stood out, and these are all safe when used appropriately. You may opt to use one or multiple of these application methods depending on your specific needs because each spans a wide range of emotional and physical wellness benefits. It could be composed of a single essential oil or a complex combination of several oils.

Aromatic

Your ability to smell is a powerful tool to elicit strong physiological, mental, and emotional reaction by your body – the aromatic approach. Essential oils' volatility enables the oils to be easily absorbed by your smell receptors that directly link, by your olfactory nerves, to your limbic system (the part of your brain that controls the function of emotions, memories, and stimulation). Diffusion is one of the simplest methods in the aromatic approach and doesn't need any special diffusing device. With just a few drops of your prepared essential oil on your palm, bring it close to your nose, and breathe deeply. Other uses of the aromatic method are for your car's air vents using a cotton ball as medium or for your furniture, carpets, or linens by mixing the essential oil in a spray bottle with water. You may also add the essential oil to your laundry batches, when you dry your sheets, or as a household surface cleaner.

Topical

Considered very effective in applying essential oils, the topical application leverages the low molecular weights of the substances in oils so your skin can easily absorb them. Once in the skin, the essential oils start to exhibit their benefits on the localized part of your body. Even as an oil, you may increase its absorbency with a light massage, which increases the blood flow in the area of application that radiates throughout your body. If you have sensitive skin, try using a carrier oil like fractionated coconut oil to avoid skin irritation. Carrier oils will dilute potent essential oils, especially if you are using the oil for the first time. The usual ratio that is used is: one part of essential oil to three parts of carrier oil. Avoid overwhelming your skin by using a large dose at once. Try several small doses throughout the day, typically every 4 to 6 hours or as needed. Since women's skin is unique from one another, the doses may vary amongst women according to their size, age, and overall health. The topical method can be used on your neck, forehead, temples, chest, abdomen, as well as your arms, legs, and feet soles. You may also add a few oil drops into a warm bath, make a hot or cold compress out of a water-soaked towel or cloth then adding the essential oil, or add it to your favorite lotion or moisturizer before applying to your skin. Just make sure to avoid the skin around your eyes and inner ears, or to a damaged, broken, or injured skin.

Internal

Essential oils have been used way back into our history. Back then, there were essential oils that were incorporated in culinary dishes and dietary supplements. Do you sprinkle cinnamon on your oatmeal? How about the soothing peppermint tea you consumed this morning? Have you tried topping your spaghetti with basil? Yes, without you knowing it, you have been infusing your food intake with these essential oils.

Aside from the flavoring and aromatic properties to foods, when in concentrated form, essential oils can be used to potently target specific health problems for optimal benefits. Once ingested, the essential oil enters your bloodstream and is transported throughout your body and just like any other food that you consume, these oils are metabolized by your liver then excreted through your feces. In coordination with your medical practitioner, take note of the proper dosage and administration of your choice of essential oil to avoid toxicity problems.

How can you leverage the internal application of essential oils? Use it when you cook or bake as substitute for dried herbs and spices. But since oils are very potent, start with small amounts. You may also use toothpick ends dipped into the essential oil instead of using drops. How about those beverages that you love? Spice your water, smoothies, milk, tea, or any other drink that you enjoy with a drop.

Step-by-Step Preparation

As mentioned earlier in this e-book, essential oils could be leveraged to support your entire endocrine system and promote the balance of your hormones. While each oil has varying application purposes, our focus is how to stabilize your estrogen dominance. Now, let's get down to business and start making those miracle workers! You can use these blends within 5 minutes of preparation time.

All-Around Oil for Today's Women Blend

Mix 10 drops each of clary sage and frankincense with 5 drops each of lavender and copaiba. Top the mix with fractionated coconut oil. As the blend suggests, it's an oil that could be used for any female related discomforts.

Bloat No More Blend

Combine 4 drops each of cypress and grapefruit with 2 drops of fennel and a tablespoon of fractionated coconut oil. Massage the blend on the area of your stomach.

Goodbye Menstrual Cramp Blend

Starting with 9 drops of lavender oil, add 4 drops each of clary sage and marjoram. Then you can top the mix with fractionated coconut oil so the blend could readily be absorbed by the skin.

Hormones and Skin Oil Serum

In a 2-ounce bottle, mix 1 ounce of evening primrose, 30 drops each of clary sage, thyme, and ylang-ylang. You can then put this mixture into a glass vial with a dropper. Rub 5 drops of this oil serum onto your neck twice daily.

Just the Right Level Serum

To have just the right levels of hormones in your system, mix 2 drops each of clary sage, frankincense, lavender, and neroli. Then add a drop of ylang-ylang. Put the mixed oils in a roller bottle then fill with fractionated coconut oil. Morning and night, roll the mix over your neck (thyroid) and along your lower back or over your kidneys (adrenals).

No More Cramps Blend

You will need 4 drops of lavender mixed with 2 drops each of clary sage and rose plus 2 teaspoons of fractionated coconut oil. Massage the mix into your abdomen area.

Red-Day Massage Blend

Start with 6 drops of lavender. Add 3 drops each of clary sage and rose. Mix this combination with 4 teaspoons of fractionated coconut oil. With this oil blend, gently rub your abdomen, back, or any part of your body for an instant relief.

Symbiotic Hormones Blend

Combine 10 drops of clary sage, 8 drops each of lavender and geranium, and 4 drops each of bergamot and ylang-ylang. Put the mixture in a rollerball bottle and top it up with fractionated coconut oil. Roll this blend over your ovaries and pulse points (neck, ankles, and wrists) for 2 to 3 times daily.

Soothe The Young Blend

When your hormones fluctuate during menstruation, PMS is triggered by the imbalance in your hormones and neurotransmitters. A simple aromatherapy formula could improve this imbalance and aid in alleviating the symptoms brought on by PMS, as well as other female hormone-related issues.

With 2 drops of clary sage, add 1 drop of geranium, and a drop of ylang-ylang. Since clary sage oil is known to promote dopamine in your brain, it helps to lift your mood together with modulating the estrogen level in your body. As to the geranium oil, it triggers the release of your adrenal hormones and reduces hormone level fluctuations.

Bath For The Young Blend

Put together 4 drops each of clary sage and bergamot, 2 drops of geranium, a drop of ylang-ylang, and ¼ cup of Epsom salt. Make sure you put salt into the mixture first before adding it into a warm bath. The salt would keep the oils from swimming on top of your bath. Plus, it will give you a magnesium boost for your bone structure.

More Than a Soak Therapeutic Blend

Combine the following – 1 cup each of sea and Epsom salts, 3 drops each of lavender and frankincense, and 2 drops of clary sage. In a small bowl, mix the two salts then add to your bath water. Blend the essential oils then add to your bath. Stir everything with your hand. Enjoy your soak for 20 minutes then rinse off in the shower. If you stay longer, you'd reabsorb the toxins. This blend intends to balance your mood and give you a good night's sleep.

Bloodfest Diffuser Blend

When you find your menstrual bleeding is more than usual, combine 10 drops of geranium and 5 drops each of helichrysum and cistus. Put the combination in a diffuser with water. Alternatively, with a drop each on both of your hands, inhale deeply three times.

Emotions Diffuser Blend

Simply mix 2 drops each of geranium, bergamot, and ylang-ylang. Put the mixture in a diffuser with water. Alternatively, put a drop each on both of your hands and take three deep breaths when your emotionally stressed. With geranium's efficacy in flushing out your unwanted emotions and bergamot's ability to even out your mood swings, this mixture would give you that feeling of serenity.

Ignite Your Passion Diffuser Blend

Combine 2 drops each of lavender and bergamot plus a drop of both ylang-ylang and vetiver for this passion-triggering formula. Add the mix to a diffuser with water. This is a very good de-stressor.

Conclusion

You are reading this e-book because one way or another, you find the importance of essential oils in addressing your hormonal imbalance; more specifically, estrogen dominance. And consequently, you've learned more, especially about the intricate functions and processes of your body. You may have been taught in school about hormones, but now that you've reached the conclusion of this e-book, you have become 'at-first-name-basis' with the hormones that greatly affect women just like you around the globe ranging from pre-teens to post-menopausal stages in their lives.

You have learned that hormones are naturally produced chemicals within your body system. Their purpose? To send important messages from one specific part of your body to another. They regulate the vital processes in your body from the simplest hunger to the more intricate function like concentration and making important decisions in your life.

As a common practice, women from all walks of life had leveraged the pharmaceutical industry when dealing with hormonal imbalance. Don't get me wrong; I'm not discounting the efficacy of these hormone-synthesized products in the market, but it also is not an exaggeration that most of the time, some of these products are so aggressive that they result to undesirable side effects.

Here is where essential oils take the lead. They are holistic and take the all-natural approach in balancing your hormones. But tons of essential oils that could stabilize your hormonal system saturate the market, both physical and virtual. Since these essential oils are powerful and strong essences and extracts, so make sure you have amply researched their usages and restrictions, as well as consulted with your health practitioner. This e-book only serves as a guide for women all around the globe who suffer the effects of having estrogen dominance.

What is the greatest point in all of these?

There is no such thing as 'too much' when your concern is doing the best you can to maintain a hormonally balanced body system. With your hormone levels well-regulated, you can live a life with more energy and maintaining a healthy weight wouldn't feel like a great struggle anymore. And last but not the least, who wouldn't want the bliss of sleep at the end of the day? Listen to what your body says and give it what it really needs.

www.ingramcontent.com/pod-product-compliance
Lightning Source LLC
Chambersburg PA
CBHW072029280526
45788CB00007B/2735